Preface

The standardized manipulation of moxibustion was drawn up by the World Federation of Acupuncture-Moxibustion Societies. In addition to the main body, there are three referential annexes, namely A, B and C; and two normative annexes, namely D and E.

Supporting institutions: Institute of Acupuncture and Moxibustion of China Academy of Chinese Medical Sciences, Anhui University of Traditional Chinese Medicine.

Main authors: Liu Weihong, Yang Jun.

Assistant authors: Han Yanjing, Wang Xiaohong, Yang Yuyang, Ma Lanping, Tan Yuansheng, Zhang Qingping, Yang Lili, Liu Wanning, Qi Shulan.

International members of the working group: Judy James (Australia), Bin Jiangwu (Canada), Liu Weihong (China), Yang Jun (China), Hsu Shengfeng (Taiwan, China), Rinaldo Rinaldi (Italia), Koo Ja Own (Korea), Arna Kausland (Norway), Lau KahYong(Singapore), Kuo Tung Ho(Singapore).

International observers: Wakayama Ikuro (Japan), Katai Shuichi (Japan).

U0307262

Introduction

"Acupuncture" and "Moxibustion" are two main therapies in acupuncture and moxibustion medicine. The scientific researches have concluded that moxibustion therapy offers unique advantages over certain diseases, especially in enhancing the function of the immune system. In view of the rapid expansion of the use of acupuncture and moxibustion worldwide, setting up the standard of the manipulation for moxibustion therapy is extremely important in order to clarify its proper application, enhance its effectiveness, and reduce or avoid its side effects.

1 Scope

This standard defines terms of the common moxibustion, specifies its procedures and requirements, operational methods, and gives precautions and contraindications of moxibustion.

This standard is applicable to the common manipulation of moxibustion.

2 Quotation Norms

The following referenced documents are indispensable for the application of this document. For dated references, only the edition cited applies. For undated references, the latest edition of the referenced document (including any amendments) applies.

Guidelines on Basic Training and Safety in Acupuncture World Health Organization (1999)

WHO International Standard Terminologies on Traditional Medicine in the Western Pacific Region World Health Organization(2007)

WHO Standard Acupuncture Point Locations in the Western Pacific Region World Health Organization(2008)

3 Terms and Definitions

The following terms and definitions are applicable to this standard.

3.1 Moxibustion

Moxibustion is a therapy which treats and prevents diseases by mainly using moxa floss. The combustion of the moxa floss permits transmission of heat to the acupoints or other parts of the body that have various pathological change. It is an external therapy to treat and/or prevent diseases and promote health of the body.

3.2 Moxa Floss

Mugwort leaves are processed to create a soft flavescent cashmere–like substance. It is rated into various grades according to its fineness. Moxa floss of high quality is usually used for direct moxibustion.

3.3 Moxa Stick

A long cigar–shaped stick is made by rolling or compressing moxa floss. These moxa sticks are sorted into two categories: pure moxa stick (no substances added) or medicated moxa stick if they contain other herbal ingredients. Smokeless moxa sticks are made with a special process to avoid producing excessive smoke while they are burning.

3.4 Moxa Cone

Moxa cone can be made by compressing, rolling or shaping the moxa floss. The machine–made ones can be cone–shaped or column–shaped. Their sizes vary from the wheat–grain size to the soybean and the jujube–stone sizes. According to the sizes they are called small cones, medium cones, and large cones, respectively.

3.5 Warm Needling Moxibustion

This technique combines acupuncture needling and moxibustion by fixing moxa floss (one section of moxa stick or a ball of moxa floss) on the top of needle handle during the retention of needles of the acupuncture treatment.

3.6 Direct Moxibustion

Direct moxibustion is the method of burning moxa cones directly on the skin. Depending on the degree of the heat stimulation to skin, it can be classified into scarring moxibustion and non–scarring moxibustion.

3.7 Indirect Moxibustion

Indirect moxibustion is performed by placing a material between the moxa cone and the skin. According to the different materials used, it can be classified as moxibustion on ginger, moxibustion on salt, moxibustion on garlic and so on.

3.8 Moxa Burner

A moxa burner is a tool specially designed for moxibustion therapy. Presently, they are commonly called moxibustion stand, moxibustion barrel, moxibustion box, moxibustion cylinder and moxibustion bowl or plate.

3.9 Fainting due to Moxibustion

Fainting due to moxibustion refers to the extreme response symptoms such as sudden dizziness, pale complexion, vertigo, nausea, sweating, palpitation, cold extremities, and a drop in the blood pressure during the moxibustion. In severe cases, there might be loss of consciousness, with stumbling, purple lips and nails, incontinence of urine and stool, profuse sweating and a weak pulse.

4 Procedures and Requirements

4.1 Preparations before Operation

4.1.1 Materials Needed

When using a moxa stick, choose a pure moxa stick or medicated moxa stick based on the state of disease and make sure that the package is intact without any mold or moisture.

When using moxa cone, choose pure moxa floss without any mold and moisture.

When using indirect moxibustion, prepare selected materials to place between the moxa cones and the skin. Check that these materials are not moldy or moisture. Make these materials into flat surface/piece with air holes of appropriate size.

When using a moxibustion burner, choose suitable one for the area for moxibustion, such as moxibustion stand, moxibustion barrel and moxibustion box.

Get the ignition tools ready, such as matches, lighters, incense threads and paper strings, etc, as well as the treatment disks, bending plates, forceps and fire extinguishing tube before starting the treatment.

4.1.2 Point Selection and Location

The selection of acupoints is based on the diagnosis and treatment plan. Select and locate the acupoints according to the disease.

The location of the acupoints should be consistent with the standard location published in the *WHO Standard Acupuncture Point Locations in the Western Pacific Region.*

4.1.3 Posture of the Body

Choose a suitable body posture which facilitates the manipulation and is also comfortable and safe for the patient during the treatment.

4.1.4 Environmental Setting Required

Be aware of environmental hygiene and avoid pollution. In order to maintain good ventilation, install ventilation facilities or air purifiers if possible.

4.1.5 Disinfection

All the disinfections mentioned above should follow the instruction on the sterilization mentioned in the *Guidelines on Basic Training and Safety in Acupuncture* published in 1999 by WHO.

4.1.5.1 Needle Disinfection

When treating with warm needling moxibustion, disposable needles should be used. If the needles are used repeatedly, they should be sterilized strictly with autoclave or other appropriate methods such as ethylene oxide gas.

4.1.5.2 Skin Disinfection

When treating with warm needling moxibustion, clean the treatment area of the skin from the center to the peripheral parts using cotton balls with medical alcohol or 0.5% ~ 1% iodophor. The area to be strongly stimulated should be sterilized by using cotton balls with 0.5% ~ 1% iodophor.

4.1.5.3 Practitioner's Disinfection

Before treating patient with warm needling moxibustion, the acupuncturists can use soapy water to wash the hands, and then clean them again using cotton balls with medical alcohol or any another sterilizer.

4.2 Operating Method

4.2.1 Moxa Stick Moxibustion

4.2.1.1 Suspended Moxibustion

The acupuncturist applies a burning moxa stick vertically above a selected point/area without touching the skin so that moderate heat can be felt on the area. The suspended heating modes of moxibustion can be gentle moxibustion, circling moxibustion and pecking sparrow moxibustion.

4.2.1.1.1 Gentle moxibustion

Ignite a moxa stick at one end and suspend it 2 ~ 3cm above the treatment area of the skin to transmit a mild warmth sensation to the area until the skin becomes slightly red without burning sensation.

4.2.1.1.2 Circling moxibustion

Ignite a moxa stick at one end and suspend it 2 ~ 3cm above the treatment area and move it in a circular motion parallel to the skin to bring mild warmth sensation to the area without burning the skin.

4.2.1.1.3 Pecking sparrow moxibustion

Ignite a moxa stick at one end and suspend it 2 ~ 3cm above the treatment area and move the stick up and down over the acupoint without touching the skin like a bird pecking a tree.

4.2.1.2 Pressing Moxibustion

Put 6 ~ 8 layers of tissue–paper, gauze or cotton cloth etc. on the treatment area and press the area using a burning moxa stick by keeping it for 1 ~ 2 seconds to bring the heat to the skin. Once the patient feels partial burning and pain, the moxa stick should be removed. Press 3 ~ 7 times at each acupoint. When the skin becomes slightly red, the moxa stick and the paper or cloth can be removed.

Pressing moxibustion usually uses medicated moxa stick. Choose the different moxa stick according to the pathology of a disease. See the Annex A.

4.2.2 Warm Needling Moxibustion

Needle the selected acupoint as usual. After the arrival of *qi* and the suitable manipulations of reinforcing or reducing, directly place a small section of the moxa stick (about 1 ~ 3cm long) on the needle handle and ignite it. Or wrap a 2 ~ 3g ball–shaped moxa floss on the needle handle and ignite it. When it burns out, remove the ashes and then the needles. A piece of cardboard would be placed on the skin around the needle to catch the ashes as they fall to avoid burning the skin.

4.2.3 Moxa Cone Moxibustion

4.2.3.1 Direct Moxibustion

Start by making an appropriate size of moxa cone with moxa of high quality to suit the patient's condition. Then place the moxa cone directly on the selected point and ignite its top. In order to fix the moxa cone on the skin, apply some adhesive or stimulus such as garlic juice, vaseline, glycerine, water, or medical alcohol before placing the moxa cone.

When 50% ~ 80% of the moxa cone has burned and the skin appears flush and burning sensation is felt, removes the moxa cone and replaces it with another one. Repeat the procedure until the required amount of cones is completed. This method involves light stimuli without scar and purulence. Hence, it is called non–scarring moxibustion, or heat sensation moxibustion.

When more than half of the moxa cone is burned and the skin flushes and burning sensation is felt, the acupuncturist can press, tap gently or scratch the skin around the buring moxa to reduce the pain sensation and distract the patient's attention. When the moxa cone is burned out, put another one until the required amount of cones is completed. This strong stimulation may lead to aseptic suppuration with scars. This method is called scarring moxibustion, diathermic moxibustion, and suppurative moxibustion. Various sizes of moxa cone for direct moxibustion are shown in the Annex D.

4.2.3.2　Indirect Moxibustion

Place a selected material on the treatment area and place a moxa cone on the material then ignite the moxa cone from its top. When the skin reddens or the heating pain is felt, lift the material with moxa cone away from the skin for a moment and replace at once. Keep doing so until the end of the treatment. For patients who need light stimuli, when 2/3 of the moxa cone has burned, remove the moxa cone or replace it with a new one until the required amount of cones is complete. For patients who need strong stimuli, when 2/3 of the moxa cone has burned, the acupuncturist can gently tap or scratch the surrounding area to distract the patient's attention and relieve the pain. When the moxa cone is burnt out, put another one until the required amount of cones is complete.

Refer to Annex B for the method of common indirect moxibustion and its preparation.

4.2.4　Moxa Burner Moxibustion

The moxa burner is used by putting moxa sticks or moxa floss into the moxa burner to start the treatment. Its advantages are convenient, safe, and comfortable.

Refer to Annex C for the common moxa burners and their usage.

4.2.4.1　Moxibustion with Moxa Stand

Insert the burning moxa stick in the moxa stand from the top and fix the stand directing on the acupoint. Acupuncturist or patient can adjust the position of moxa stick in order to regulate the temperature suitable to the patient's tolerance. After the treatment, remove the moxa stand and take out the moxa stick. Then put out the fire and clean up the ashes.

4.2.4.2　Moxibustion with Moxa Barrel

Firstly take out the inner barrel to put the moxa floss into it and replace the inner barrel. Then ignite the moxa floss and place the moxibustion barrel outdoor. Wait until the smoke becomes less and the exterior surface of outer barrel becomes hot. Bring it back indoor and put a lid on it. Arrange the patient in an appropriate posture and place the moxa barrel on the appropriate chosen area over 8 ~ 10 layers of cotton cloth and gauze. Have the patient feel a comfortable level of heat without burning the skin. After the treatment, remove the moxa barrel and put out the fire and clean up the ashes.

4.2.4.3　Moxibustion with Moxa Box

Place the moxa box on the moxibustion area of the body. Prepare suitable moxa floss or moxa stick according to the required treatment time. Ignite moxa floss or moxa stick on the iron gauze which is in the lower part of the box and place the lid on top. Have the patient feel comfortable warmth without a burning sensation. The skin flushes. If patient has a burning sensation, open the lid or slightly lift up the moxa box away from skin for a short while, and then place it down again. Keep doing so repeatedly until the required amount of cones is complete. After the treatment, remove the moxa box, put out the fire and clean up the ashes.

4.2.4.4 Moxibustion with Moxa Bowl or Plate

Ignite the moxa floss and put it into a ceramic bowl or plate. When the bottom of the bowl or plate is hot enough, place it over 8 ~ 10 pieces of gauze or cotton on the treatment area. The heat should be felt comfortable by the patient and never burn the skin. After the treatment, remove the instrument, put out the fire and clean up the ashes.

4.2.4.5 Moxibustion with Moxa Cylinder

Ignite the incense stick and put it into the moxa cylinder. When the head of the cylinder is heated, place it on the layers of gauze or cotton on the treatment area. The heat should be felt comfortable by the patient and make the skin become red without burning the skin. After the treatment, remove the incense stick, put out the fire and clean up the ashes.

4.3 Post-Moxibustion Disposition

After moxibustion, the skin will appear red and hot. No special care is needed since the redness will gradually disappear on its own.

If skin is burned, edema or blistering will occur. Blisters of about 1cm in diameter can be gradually absorbed by the body without any treatment. Larger blisters can be removed by sterilized scissors or punctured by sterilized needles to remove the fluid. Then an anti-inflammatory ointment can be applied to it. There is no need to remove the pus since the scab will form soon. Blistered skin can scab within 5 ~ 8 days, and the scab will fall off without any scar left.

Scarring moxibustion will damage the basal layer of skin which will cause edema, ulceration, fluid exudation, and even form abscesses. Light damages only destroy the basal layer of skin. Damaged skin will scab within 7 ~ 20 days and the scab will fall off, leaving a permanent light scar. Heavy damages will destroy the dermis tissues. Damaged skin will scab with a thick crust and the scab will fall off within 20 ~ 50 days, leaving a permanent thick scar, which is called moxibustion sores. When the moxibustion sores are festering, the patient should not be engaged in heavy work and need to rest well to prevent infection. If infection, mild redness or swelling appears, disinfection and anti-inflammatory treatment around the moxibustion sores is needed. Generally, these symptoms will disappear in a short period of time. If swelling and burning pain are severe, the patient can take oral or external anti-inflammatory medication. If the suppurative parts are comparatively deep, a surgeon's assistance is needed. The acupuncturist must abide by the law of his/her country when engaging in the scarring moxibustion procedure.

5 Precautions

5.1 In order for the patients to gradually get accustomed to moxibustion the heating intensity of moxibustion fire should start with low heat then high heat; the amount/number of moxibustion should be fewer at beginning then increase. The degree of moxibustion should start from mild to more intensive. Refer to Annex D for the amount, time and course of moxibustion treatment.

5.2 Scarring moxibustion should be performed according to the law and with consent of the patients who have understood the process of the therapy thoroughly.

5.3 The body hair should be shaved off if there is too much on the site of moxibustion. The consent of the patients is needed.

5.4 Before treatment, explain the situation that may arise to the patient. Special care should be taken for moxibustion patients with unclear consciousness, sensory disturbances, mental confusion, local circulatory disorders and diabetes.

5.5 Management needs to be done after the direct moxibustion to prevent infection. For example, avoiding water, and keeping the treatment area clean.

5.6 Be aware of the occurrence of fainting due to moxibustion. If it occurs, see Annex E for the management methods.

5.7 Do not treat patients when they feel nervous, hungry, sweaty (dehydrated) and fatigued.

5.8 Be cautious of the occurrence of falling ash and moxa cones which may burn the skin or the clothes. When moxibustion treatment is finished, the rest of moxa stick should be put out to prevent its burning elsewhere. Clean up any fallen ashes onto the bed to avoid damage to beddings.

5.9 When moxibustion is used on infants, the acupuncturist should put his/her index and middle fingers of one hand beside the site of moxibustion to experience the temperature of the heat to avoid burning the skin of the infants.

6 Contraindications

6.1 Scarring moxibustion is forbidden on the face, regio colli anterior, precordium, joints and tendon, nipples, genitals, part with superficial great vessel, affected skin, and acutely-inflamed part. Direct moxibustion is also forbidden on nipples and genitals.

6.2 Patients with symptoms such as heat-stroke and hypertensive crisis, late-phase tuberculosis with plenty of hemoptysis are not suitable for moxibustion treatment.

6.3 Scarring moxibustion on the lumbosacral and lower abdominal areas is to be avoided during pregnancy.

Annex A
(Informative)
Common Moxa Sticks

A.1   Pure Moxa Stick

A.1.1   Common Pure Moxa Stick

Take 20 ~ 30g of pure moxa floss and wrap it with paper into cylinder shape(Figure A1).

A.1.2   Compressed Moxa Stick

Take 6 ~ 10g of pure moxa floss and compress it into a paper tube of 8 ~ 10cm long and 2 ~ 3cm in diameter. Expose the moxa floss out of paper tube when use it(Figure A2).

A.1.3   Incense Moxa Stick

Grind the mugwort, add some adhesive agent, and press it into a thin solid stick. The stick is similar to an incense thread. It is usually used with the moxa cylinder (Figure A3).

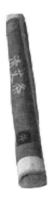

Figure A1   Common Pure Moxa Stick

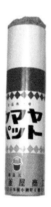

Figure A2   Compressed Moxa Stick

A.2   Smokeless Moxa Stick

Heat the moxa stick fully and make it carbonized. The carbonized stick is called smokeless moxa stick. Its usage is similar to the common pure moxa stick. (Figure A4)

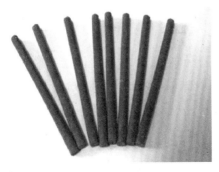

Figure A3   Incense Moxa Stick

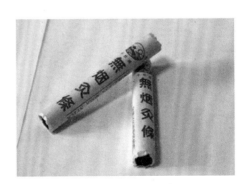

Figure A4   Smokeless Moxa Stick

A.3 Commonly-used Medicated Moxa Stick

Medicated moxa stick is made by mixing Chinese herb ingredients into the pure moxa stick. Grind equal amount of bark of Chinese cassia tree, dried ginger, common aucklandia root, angelica, wildginger, dahurian angelica root, Chinese atractylodes, common myrrh tree, frankincense, xanthoxylum piperitum into a powder. Mix the powder with the moxa floss and use 6g of the powder per stick.Medicated moxa stick is much stronger in its pungent and warm properties and has a greater penetrating function when compared with the pure moxa stick. It is commonly used for intractable deficiency cold diseases.

A.4 *Taiyi* Moxa Stick Moxibustion

A special moxa roll made of sandalwood, notopterygium rhizome, cassia twig, dahurian angelica root and other Chinese medicinal herbs, used for the treatment of wind-cold-dampness arthralgia, abdominal pain of cold type and dysmenorrhea.

A.5 Thunder-fire Wonder Moxibustion

A type of medicinal moxa roll using Chinese eagle wood, common aucklandia root, frankincense and other Chinese medicinal herbs to treat diseases such as cold and pain in the epigastrium and abdomen, rheumatism and dysmenorrhea.

Annex B
(Informative)
Common Indirect Moxibustion

B.1 Moxibustion on Ginger

Slice fresh ginger into flat pieces with a diameter about 2 ~ 3cm and 0.4 ~ 0.6cm in thickness. Pierce several holes in the slice of ginger with a needle. Put the ginger slice on the acupoints or diseased areas, then place moxa cone on the slice and light the cone. When the cone burns out, replace it with another one until completion of treatment. The skin must become red but should not appear burned when completion. This method is frequently used in case of vomiting, abdominal pain, diarrhea and pain due to cold.

B.2 Moxibustion on Garlic

Slice fresh garlic seeds into pieces of about 0.3 ~ 0.5cm in thickness and pierce several holes in the slices with a needle. Put a garlic slice on the acupoint or diseased area, then place a moxa cone on the slice and light it. When the cone burns out, replace it with another one until completion of treatment. This method is frequently used in case of scrofula, tuberculosis and the early stage of pyogenic infection and painful swelling.

B.3 Moxibustion on Salt

Apply clean salt in the navel or put a slice of ginger on salt. The size of the moxa cone is bigger than the ones used in other moxibustion method in this case. The moxa cone needs to be replaced once they burned out. Repeat the procedure until the end of the treatment. This method is frequently used for *Yin* syndromes of exogenous febrile disease, simultaneous vomiting and diarrhea and depletion due to apoplexy.

B.4 Moxibustion on Monkshood-cake

Monkhood cake is 2 ~ 3cm in diameter and 0.5 ~ 0.8cm in thickness. It is made of powdered aconite mixed with wine. Pierce the cake to make several holes with a needle. Place the cake on the acupoint or diseased area, then place a moxa cone on the cake and light it. When the cone burns out, replace it with another one until completion of treatment. This method is frequently used in case of impotence and prospermia caused by insufficiency of the kidney-*yang* and chronic ulcerations of sores and ulcers.

B.5 Moxibustion on Pepper-cake

Make a pancake that is 2 ~ 3cm in diameter and 0.5 ~ 0.8cm in thickness made of white pepper powder, flour and water. Put some of powdered Chinese medicines at the center of the cake: lilac, bark of Chinese cassia tree, artificial musk. Place the pepper-cake on the acupoint or diseased area, place a moxa cone and light it. When the cone burns out, replace it with another one until completion of treatment. This method is frequently used in case of paralysis, pain and partial numbness caused by rheumatism.

B.6 Moxibustion on Bean-cake

Make a cake of yellow rice wine and brown bean powder of 2 ~ 3cm in diameter and 0.5 ~ 0.8cm in thickness. Pierce several holes in the cake with a needle. Place a bean–cake on the acupoint or diseased area, place a moxa cone on the cake and light it. When the cone burns out, replace it with another one until completion of treatment. This method is frequently used in case of carbuncle and gangrene on back at the early stage or chronic ulcerations.

Annex C
(Informative)
Common Moxa Burner

C.1 Moxibustion Stand

It is a specially–designed plastic or wooden tool which is either barrel or trapezoid shaped with all sides hollowed. On the top there are round holes to place and fix the moxa sticks. There is an iron gauze in the lower middle part about 3 ~ 4cm from the bottom of the stand and there are two small rings at the both sides. A rubber belt and a fire extinguishing tube are provided. Position the lighted moxa stick into the hole on the top where it can be moved. Place the stand on acupoint with the rubber belt and raise or lower moxa sticks to adjust the temperature. The patients should feel a little hot but no pain. After the treatment, the remaining burning head of the moxa sticks should be removed into the tube to extinguish the fire. Figure C1 ~ C3 for common moxibustion stands.

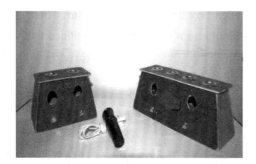

Figure C1   Trapezoid Shaped Stand

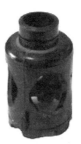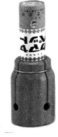

Figure C2   Barrel Shaped Stand

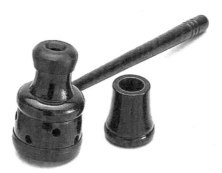

Figure C3   Stand with a Handle

C.2 Moxibustion Barrel

This moxibustion barrel is made of either iron or copper about 2 ~ 5mm in thickness and consists of an inner and outer barrel. There are holes at the bottoms and on the walls of the inner and outer barrels. There is also a removable lid which fit in the outer barrel. A stand affixed to the inner barrel keeps a distance with the outer barrel and a handle on the outer barrel is convenient for holding. Fill the moxa floss in the inner barrel and light it then place the inner barrel into the outer one and cover with the lid (Figure C4).

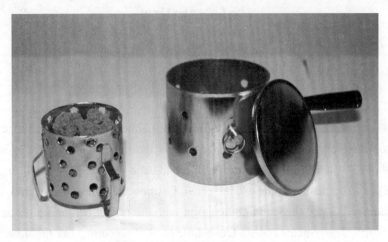

Figure C4　Moxibustion Barrel

C.3　Moxibustion Box

It is a specially–designed rectangular bottomless wooden box with a removable lid. There is a piece of iron gauze in the lower middle part about 4 ~ 6cm from the bottom edge of the box. Place the box on an acupoint or diseased area, and then add lighted moxa floss or moxa sticks on the gauze, and cover with the lid (Figure C5).

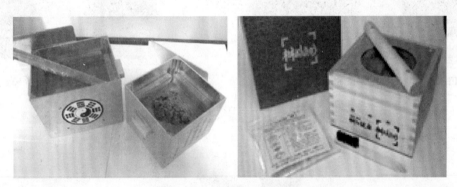

Figure C5　Moxibustion Box

C.4　Moxa Cone Apparatus

It is a specific metal round tool about 6cm in diameter and 2cm in height which is hollow inside without a bottom. There are several round holes on the top surface to position the moxa cones. These cones will be burned simultaneously during the moxibustion treatment. The moxa cone apparatus can be held or put on the acupoint (Figure C6).

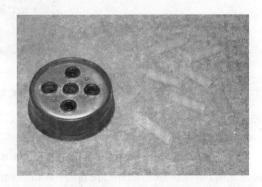

Figure C6　Moxa Cone Apparatus and Moxa Cones

C.5　Moxibustion with Cardboard Base

Roll moxa floss with a paper 4 ~ 10mm in width and 7 ~ 12mm in length. Make the cardboard base 15 ~ 35mm in diameter, 2 ~ 5mm in thickness with a small vent hole at the center. Affix the moxa roll vertically in the center. When giving the treatment, attach the cardboard to the skin with the adhesive glue on the bottom of the cardboard. The glue also prevents the moxa from falling and burning the skin. The vent in the center of cardboard allows the heat transmission. The heat intensity of the moxa can be controlled by adjusting the thickness of the cardboard used as well as the diameter of moxa roll and the grade of moxa floss(Figure C7 and C8).

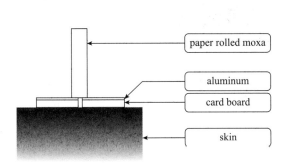

Figure C7　Diagram of Cardboard Base Type Moxibustion

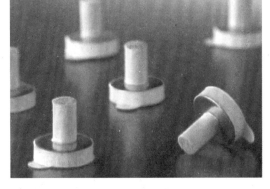

Figure C8　Cardboard Base Type Moxibustion

C.6　Moxibustion with Moxa Tube

Place about 0.1g of moxa floss on the head of a paper tube of about 7 ~ 10mm in diameter and 10 ~ 15mm in height. Attach the paper tube to the skin with the adhesive glue under the paper tube. The glue also prevents the moxa from falling and burning the skin. While the moxa floss is ignited, the heat transmits inside the tube to reach the skin. The heat produced by moxa can be controlled by adjusting the diameter of paper tube and selecting the proper grade of moxa floss(Figure C9 and C10).

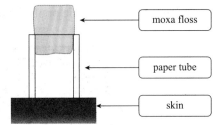

Figure C9　Diagram of Moxa Tube

Type Moxibustion

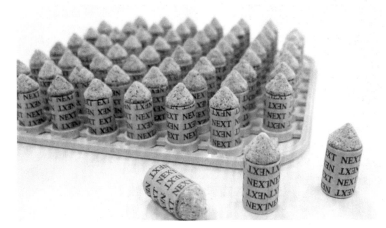

Figure C10　Moxa Tube Type Moxibustion

C.7 Moxibustion Bowl or Plate

Moxibustion bowl or plate is a ceramic round bowl or plate which warms up when holding burning moxa floss. The bowl has the cover with small holes, the plate does not have. The heat intensity varies according to the thickness of the ceramic and can be adjusted by increasing or decreasing the pieces of gauze or cotton laid between the heated skin area and the bowl or plate(Figure C11).

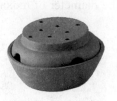 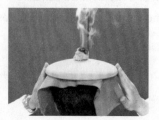

Figure C11 Moxibustion Bowl and Moxibustion Plate

C.8 Moxibustion Cylinder

This is a handy sized moxibustion tool held in the hand with a wooden handle and metallic tip. Place the burning incense stick or pure moxa stick into the cylinder from the wooden handle. Fix the burning stick at a particular point inside so that it does not reach the bottom of metallic tip. Place it on the skin or lay some pieces of gauze or cotton on the heated area below the cylinder bottom in order to regulate the temperature if necessary. After the treatment, turn the cylinder upside down to remove the stick and put out the fire. Some cylinders are made of ceramic or other materials (Figure C12).

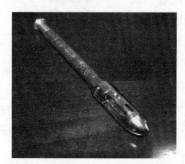 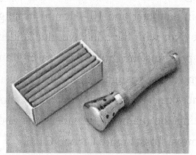

Figure C12   Moxibustion Cylinder and Incense Moxa Stick

Annex D

(Normative)

Amount of Moxa, Treatment Time and Course

D.1 Amount of Moxa

The amount of moxa used in the treatment is related to the dosage of warmth needed in the treatment. Different amount of moxa will have different efficacy. The amount of moxibustion used in moxa cone is calculated according to the size and the number of cones. The small size of the cone and the fewer cones account for the smaller amount and vice versa. The amount of moxibustion used in moxa stick or with a burner is measured by the time of the treatment. The longer the treatment is, more moxibustions are needed. The amount of pressing moxibustion is measured by the frequency of pressing. The more frequent the pressing is, the more amount of moxibustion is considered.

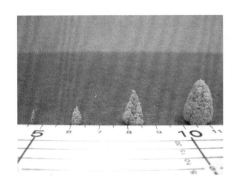

D.2 Common Sizes of Moxa Cones

The temperature will differ depending the size of moxa cones. Generally, an extremely small cone is as thin as a thread. A small cone is about 2 ~ 5mm in diameter and 4 ~ 8mm in height. A medium cone is about 6 ~ 10mm in diameter and 9 ~ 13mm in height. A large cone is about 11 ~ 15mm in diameter and 14 ~ 25mm in height. See Figure D1 for the common sizes of moxa cones.

Figure D1   Common Sizes of Moxa Cones

D.3 The Amount of Moxa Used for Various Treated Areas, Diseases and Patient's Constitution

Generally speaking, the amount of moxa will vary according to the different treated areas, diseases and patient's constitution.

For example, a small amount of moxa is suggested on areas such as the head, face, chest and the end of the extremities since the skin is thin and there are more bones and fewer muscles. On the other hand, a large amount of moxa is suggested on the waist, abdomen, shoulders, and thighs, where both the skin and muscles are thick.

The disease situation also has to do with the amount of moxa used in the treatment. For example, a large amount of moxa is effective on obstinately cold disease and *yang qi* depletion. On the other hand, a small amount of moxa is used for cold diseases, carbuncle, gangrene, numbness and pain.

The patient's constitution is another consideration. The stronger patient sustains more amount of moxa during the treatment. For weak, senior, or very young patients, a smaller amount is used in treatment.

D.4 Time and Course of Moxibustion

Time used in moxibustion treatment depends on the disease and patients, may vary from 10 to 40 minutes per treatment and 5 to 15 treatments constitute a course of treatment.

In direct moxibustion, an interval of 1 ~ 10 days between two treatments is considered depending on the diseases and patients.

Annex E
(Normative)
Management of Fainting due to Moxibustion

If a patient faints due to moxibustion, treatment should be stopped immediately. Have the patient lie down and stay warm. Most patients can recover after resting for a short while or after drinking some hot water. Stimulation at Shuigou (GV26), Neiguan (PC6) and Zusanli (ST36) may help recover. If the patients don't recover, treat as syncope. If the symptoms persist, it is necessary to refer to professional doctor. The acupuncturist must follow the law of his/her country when engaging in the above mentioned manipulation of moxibustion.

前　言

艾灸操作规范由世界针灸学会联合会制定。除了主体部分，本标准附录 A、附录 B 和附录 C 是资料性附录，附录 D 和附录 E 是规范性附录。

支持单位：中国中医科学院针灸研究所、安徽中医药大学。

主要作者：刘炜宏、杨骏。

参与者：韩焱晶、王晓红、杨宇洋、马兰萍、谭源生、张庆萍、杨立丽、刘婉宁、齐淑兰。

国际工作组成员：Judy James（澳大利亚），Bin Jiangwu（加拿大），Liu Weihong（中国），Yang Jun（中国），Hsu Shengfeng（中国台湾地区），Rinaldo Rinaldi（意大利），Koo Ja Own（韩国），Arna Kausland（挪威），Lau KahYong（新加坡），Kuo Tung Ho（新加坡）。

国际观察员：Wakayama Ikuro（日本），Katai Shuichi（日本）。

引　言

　　"针刺"和"艾灸"是针灸学中并行的两大疗法，追溯历史，灸法应该比针刺的使用历史更长。现代科学研究证实，灸法对某些疾病的疗效优于针刺，尤其是在提高机体免疫力方面有着独特的优势。规范艾灸技术操作，对于提高灸法的疗效，避免或减少对机体的损伤，推广艾灸疗法有着十分重要的意义。

1 范围

本标准规定了常用艾灸疗法的术语和定义、操作步骤与要求、操作方法、注意事项与禁忌。

本标准适用于常用艾灸技术操作。

2 规范性引用文件

下列文件对于本标准的应用是必不可少的。凡是注明日期的引用文件，说明仅该版本适用于本标准。凡是不注明日期的引用文件，说明其最新版本（包括所有的修改文件）适用于本标准。

《针灸基础培训与安全规范》 世界卫生组织（1999）

《世界卫生组织西太平洋地区传统医学术语标准》 世界卫生组织（2007）

《世界卫生组织西太平洋地区针灸穴位定位标准》 世界卫生组织（2008）

3 术语和定义

下列术语和定义适用于本技术操作规范。

3.1 艾灸

艾灸，指用艾绒或以艾绒为主要成分制成的灸材，点燃后悬置或放置在穴位或病变部位，进行烧灼、温熨，借灸火的热力以及药物的作用，达到治病、防病和保健目的的一种外治方法。

3.2 艾绒

艾绒，指艾叶经加工制成的淡黄色、细软的绒状物。根据质量优劣，可分为不同等级。质量好的艾绒可以用于直接灸。

3.3 艾条

艾条，指以艾绒为主要成分，用纸卷成的圆柱形条状物。根据内含药物的有无，分为药艾条和清艾条。经过特殊处理，使艾条在燃烧过程中很少产生烟雾，称为无烟艾条。

3.4 艾炷

艾炷，指用艾绒制作成的小圆锥形物体。每燃 1 个艾炷，称为灸 1 壮。艾炷的大小有不同，如麦粒大、黄豆大、枣核大，分别称为小壮、中壮、大壮。

3.5 温针灸

温针灸，指毫针针刺留针时，在针柄上置以艾绒或艾条段施灸的方法。

3.6 直接灸

直接灸是将艾炷直接放在穴位皮肤上施灸的方法。根据对皮肤刺激程度不同，可分为化脓灸法和非化脓灸法。

3.7 间接灸

间接灸是在艾炷与皮肤之间垫隔适当的中药材而施灸的一种方法。根据选用中药材的不同，又分为不同的间接灸，如隔姜灸、隔盐灸、隔蒜灸等。

3.8 温灸器

温灸器，指专门用于施灸的器具。目前临床常用的温灸器有灸架、灸筒和灸盒等。

3.9 晕灸

晕灸，指患者在接受艾灸治疗过程中发生晕厥的现象，表现为突然出现头晕目眩、面色苍白、恶心呕吐、汗出、心慌、四肢发凉、血压下降等症状。重者出现神志昏迷、跌仆、唇甲青紫、二便失禁、大汗、四肢厥逆、脉微欲绝。

4 操作步骤与要求

4.1 施术前准备

4.1.1 灸材选择

采用艾条灸时，应选择无霉变潮湿、包装无破损、符合病证需要的清艾条或药艾条。

采用艾炷灸时，应选择无霉变、无潮湿的清艾绒。

采用间接灸时，应准备好需要的药材，检查药材有无变质、发霉、潮湿，并制成符合治疗需要的大小、形状、平整度、孔眼等。

采用温灸器灸时，应选择合适的温灸器具，如灸架、灸筒、灸盒等。

其他辅助用具：点火工具、治疗盘、镊子、灭火管。

4.1.2 穴位选择及定位

穴位的选择，依据病种和证型选取适当的穴位或治疗部位。

穴位的定位，应符合《世界卫生组织西太平洋地区针灸穴位定位标准》的规定。

4.1.3 体位选择

施灸前，选好穴位后，应选择正确的施灸体位。要选择患者舒适、安全、能坚持施灸的全过程，医者便于操作的治疗体位。

4.1.4 环境要求

应注意治疗室的清洁卫生，避免污染；为保持良好的通风，应安装通风设备；有条件的地方，可安装空气净化设备。

4.1.5 消毒

采用温针灸针刺时，应严格消毒。医者手的清洁、针刺部位消毒、针具消毒，应符合《针灸基础培训与安全规范》。

4.1.5.1 针具消毒

应选择一次性针具。反复使用的针具可选择高压蒸汽消毒法消毒。

4.1.5.2 部位消毒

部位消毒，可用含 75% 医用乙醇或 0.5%~1% 碘伏的棉球在施术部位由中心向外做环行擦拭。

4.1.5.3 术者消毒

医者双手可用肥皂水清洗干净，再用含 75% 医用乙醇棉球擦拭，或喷抹其他消毒剂。

4.2 施术方法

4.2.1 艾条灸

4.2.1.1 悬起灸法

术者将点燃的艾条垂直悬于选定的穴位或区域上，不使艾条燃着端接触皮肤，以局部感到温热舒适为度。悬起灸分为温和灸、回旋灸、雀啄灸。

4.2.1.1.1 温和灸

术者手持艾条，将艾条的一端点燃，直接悬于施灸部位上距皮肤 2~3cm 处，灸至患者有温热舒适的感觉，无灼痛，皮肤稍有红晕。

4.2.1.1.2 回旋灸

术者手持艾条，将艾条燃着端悬于施灸部位上距皮肤 2~3cm 处，平行往复回旋熏灸，使皮肤有温热感而不至于灼痛。

4.2.1.1.3 雀啄灸

术者手持艾条，将艾条燃着端悬于施灸部位上距皮肤 2~3cm 处，对准穴位，上下移动，一起一落，忽近忽远，犹如鸟雀啄食样。

4.2.1.2 实按灸法

在施灸部位上铺设 6~8 层绵纸、纱布、绸布或棉布。术者手持艾条，将艾条的一端点燃，艾条燃着端对准施灸部位直按其上，停 1~2 秒钟，使热力透达皮肤深部。待患者感到灼烫、疼痛即移开艾条。反复点按，每次治疗时每穴可按 3~7 次。灸毕，移开纸或布，以皮肤红晕为度。

实按灸一般使用的是药艾条、太乙神针或雷火神针，可根据不同的病证选用不同的艾条，参见附录 A。

4.2.2 温针灸

先在选定的腧穴上针刺，毫针刺入穴位得气并施行适当的补泻手法，留针时将 1 ~ 3cm 长的艾条段直接插在针柄上，从底部点燃；或将 2 ~ 3g 艾绒包裹于毫针针柄顶端，捏紧成团状，点燃艾绒，待艾条段或艾绒燃尽，至无热度后除去灰烬。艾灸结束，将针取出。为防止灸治过程中艾灰脱落而灼伤皮肤，可在针灸针贴近皮肤处垫一硬纸，接住落灰。

4.2.3 艾炷灸

4.2.3.1 直接灸法

首先，将艾炷放在所选的穴位上，自艾炷尖端点燃。为便于固定，可以先在穴位皮肤上涂抹一些增加黏附或刺激作用的液汁，如大蒜汁、凡士林、甘油等，然后将艾炷黏贴其上，以加强艾炷的附着力。

在艾炷燃烧过半，或燃烧大部分（50% ~ 80%），局部皮肤潮红、灼痛时，医生即用镊子移去艾炷，更换另一艾炷，连续灸足应灸的壮数。这种灸法刺激量轻，灸后不引起化脓，不留瘢痕，称为非化脓灸法（无瘢痕灸）、透热灸、知热灸。

在艾炷燃烧过半，局部皮肤潮红、灼痛时，医生用手在施灸穴位的周围轻轻拍打或抓挠，以分散患者的注意力，减轻施灸时的痛苦。待艾炷燃毕，即以另一艾炷黏上，继续燃烧，直至灸足应灸的壮数。这种灸法刺激量重，局部组织经灸灼后产生无菌性化脓（灸疮）并留有瘢痕，称为化脓灸法（瘢痕灸）、打脓灸。不同类型的艾灸，所需艾灸的柱数不同，详细参考附录D。

4.2.3.2 间接灸法

将选定的中药材放施灸处，再把艾炷放在药材上，自艾炷尖端点燃。待艾炷燃烧至局部皮肤潮红、患者有痛觉时，将药材稍许上提，离开皮肤片刻，旋即放下，再行灸治，反复进行。需刺激量轻者，在艾炷燃至 2/3 时即移去艾炷，或更换另一艾炷续灸，直至灸足应灸的壮数；需刺激量重者，在艾炷燃至 2/3 时，医者可用手在施灸穴位的周围轻轻拍打或抓挠，以分散患者的注意力，减轻施灸时的痛苦，待艾炷燃毕，再更换另一艾炷续灸，直至灸足应灸的壮数。

常用的间接灸及其材料制备方法见附录B。

4.2.4 温灸器灸

将艾条或艾绒放入温灸器内施灸，具有使用方便、安全、舒适、节省人力的特点。

常用的温灸器具及其使用方法见附录C。

4.2.4.1 灸架灸法

将艾条点燃后插入灸架顶孔，对准穴位固定好灸架。医者或患者可通过上下调整艾条的高度以调节温度，以患者感到温热略烫、可耐受为宜。灸毕，移去灸架，取出艾条并熄灭。

4.2.4.2 灸筒灸法

首先，取出灸筒的内筒，装入艾绒后安上外筒，点燃内筒中的艾绒，放置室外，待灸筒外面热烫而艾烟较少时，盖上顶盖取回。在施灸部位上预放置 8 ~ 10 层棉布或纱布，将灸筒放在棉布上，以患者感到舒适、热力足而不烫伤皮肤为宜。灸毕，移去灸筒，取出灸艾并熄灭灰烬。

4.2.4.3 灸盒灸法

将灸盒安放于施灸部位的中央，视治疗时间取用合适的艾段或艾绒，点燃艾条段或艾绒后，置放于灸盒内中下部的铁纱上，盖上盒盖。灸至患者有温热舒适无灼痛的感觉、皮肤稍有红晕为度。如患者感到灼烫，可略掀开盒盖或抬起灸盒，使之离开皮肤片刻，旋即放下，再行灸治，反复进行，直至灸足应灸的量。灸毕，移去灸盒，取出灸艾并熄灭灰烬。

4.2.4.4 灸碗或灸盘灸法

将艾绒点燃，置于陶瓷碗或盘中。在施灸部位上预放置 8 ~ 10 层棉布或纱布。当碗或盘的顶部足够热时，放在预处理后的施灸部位。以患者感到舒适、热力足而不烫伤皮肤为宜。灸毕，移去灸碗或盘，取出艾绒并熄灭灰烬。

4.2.4.5 灸缸灸法

点燃艾绒并置于灸缸内，在施灸部位放置多层棉布或纱布。当灸缸的顶部热烫时，将其放置在预处理后的施灸部位，以患者感到舒适、热力足而不烫伤皮肤为宜。灸毕，移去灸缸，取出艾绒并熄灭灰烬。

4.3 施术后处理

施灸后，皮肤多有红晕和灼热感，不需处理，可自行消失。

灸后如对表皮基底层以上的皮肤组织造成灼伤，可发生水肿或水疱。如水疱直径在1cm左右，一般不需做任何处理，待其自行吸收即可；如水疱较大，可用消毒针刺破疱皮，放出水疱内容物，并用消毒剪剪去疱皮，暴露被破坏的基底层，涂搽消炎膏药以防止感染，创面的无菌脓液不必清理，直至结痂自愈。灸疮处皮肤可在5~8天内结痂并自动脱落，愈后一般不留瘢痕。

瘢痕灸后有时会破坏皮肤基底层或真皮组织，发生水肿、溃烂、体液渗出，甚至形成无菌性化脓。轻者仅破坏皮肤基底层，受损伤的皮肤在7~20天内结痂并自动脱落，留有永久性浅在瘢痕；重者真皮组织被破坏，创面在20~50天结厚痂并自动脱落，愈后留有永久性瘢痕，即形成灸疮。在灸疮化脓期间，不宜从事体力劳动，要注意休息，严防感染。若发生感染，如轻度发红或红肿，可在局部做消炎处理，一般短时间内可消失；如出现红肿热痛且范围较大的，在上述处理的同时口服或外用消炎药物；化脓部位较深的，应请外科医生处理。艾灸师必须遵守自己所在国家关于瘢痕灸的相关规定。

5 注意事项

5.1 施灸时，艾灸火力应先小后大，灸量先少后多，患者感觉先轻后重，以使患者逐渐适应。艾灸具体灸量、艾灸治疗时间及疗程，参见附录D。

5.2 需采用瘢痕灸时，必须先征得患者同意，并且使其对此疗法有充分的了解。

5.3 在体毛较多的部位施灸时，需剃去毛发，应事先征得患者的同意。

5.4 在艾灸前，向患者解释清楚可能发生的状况。患者如伴有意识不清、感觉障碍、精神错乱、局部循环障碍，或患有糖尿病，施灸时应特别注意。

5.5 直接灸时，操作部位应注意预防感染，如避免沾水、保持治疗部位洁净。

5.6 注意晕灸的发生。如发生晕灸现象，处理办法参见附录E。

5.7 患者在精神紧张、大汗后、劳累后或饥饿时，不适宜应用本疗法。

5.8 注意防止艾灰脱落或艾炷倾倒而烫伤皮肤或烧坏衣被。艾条灸毕后，应将剩下的艾条套入灭火管内或将燃头浸入水中，以彻底熄灭，防止再燃。如有艾灰脱落床上，应清扫干净，以免复燃。

5.9 对婴幼儿施灸时，医者应将另一手的食指、中指垫在施灸部位旁，体会热度，以免发生烫伤。

6 禁忌

6.1 颜面、心前区、大血管部和关节、肌腱处，不可用瘢痕灸；乳头、外生殖器官，不宜直接灸。

6.2 部分疾病如中暑、高血压危象、肺结核晚期大量咯血等，不宜使用艾灸疗法。

6.3 妊娠期妇女腰骶部和少腹部，不宜用瘢痕灸。

附　录　A
（资料性附录）
常用艾条

A.1　纯艾条
A.1.1　清艾条
取纯净艾绒 20 ~ 30g，用绵皮纸等包裹，卷成圆柱形长条（图 A1）。
A.1.2　压缩艾条
取 6 ~ 10g 清艾绒，将其压缩进长 8 ~ 10cm、直径 2 ~ 3cm 的纸管内。当需要使用时，将艾绒从中取出（图 A2）。

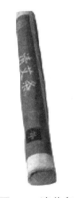

图 A1　清艾条

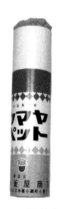

图 A2　压缩艾条

A.1.3　香艾条
将艾蒿磨碎，添加黏附剂，将它们压缩进固体细小管内。此艾灸条和线香一样，通常放在灸缸中使用（图 A3）。
A.2　无烟艾条
将艾条加热，使其碳化。被碳化的艾条叫作无烟艾条，它和清艾条的使用方法一样（图 A4）。

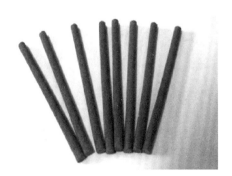

图 A3　香艾条

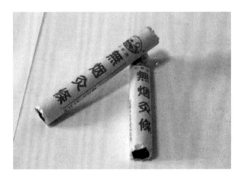

图 A4　无烟艾条

A.3　普通药艾条

药艾条是指将中药与清艾条混合。取肉桂、干姜、木香、独活、细辛、白芷、苍术、没药、乳香、川椒各等份，研成细末。将药末混入艾绒中，每支艾条加药末 6g。药艾条较清艾条辛温通透之力更强，一般用于顽固性虚寒之疾。

A.4　太乙神针（太乙药条）

太乙神针为一种特别的艾灸卷，由檀香木、羌活、桂枝、白芷粉末以及其他的中药制成。一般用于风寒湿痹、寒性腹痛、痛经。

A.5　雷火神针

雷火神针为一种药用艾灸卷，由沉香、木香、乳香以及其他的中药制成。一般用于上腹痛、腹痛、风湿病、痛经等。

附　录　B

（资料性附录）

常用间接灸

B.1　隔姜灸

用鲜姜切成直径2~3cm、厚0.4~0.6cm的薄片，中间以针刺数孔，然后置于应灸的腧穴部位或患处，再将艾炷放在姜片上点燃施灸。当艾炷燃尽，易炷再灸，直至灸完应灸的壮数。治疗完毕，皮肤潮红，但没有灼伤。常用于治疗因寒而致的呕吐、腹痛、腹泻及风寒痹痛等。

B.2　隔蒜灸

用鲜大蒜头切成厚0.3~0.5cm的薄片，中间以针刺数孔，然后置于应灸腧穴部位或患处，再将艾炷放在蒜片上点燃施灸。当艾炷燃尽，易炷再灸，直至灸完应灸的壮数。此法多用于治疗瘰疬、肺结核及初起的肿疡等。

B.3　隔盐灸

用纯净的食盐填敷于脐部，或于盐上再置一薄姜片，上置大艾炷施灸。当艾炷燃尽，易炷再灸，直至灸完应灸的壮数。此法多用于治疗伤寒阴证或吐泻并作、中风脱证等。

B.4　隔附子饼灸

将附子研成粉末，用酒调和，做成直径2~3cm、厚0.5~0.8cm的薄饼，中间以针刺数孔，然后置于应灸腧穴部位或患处，再将艾炷放在附子饼上点燃施灸。当艾炷燃尽，易炷再灸，直至灸完应灸的壮数。此法多用于治疗命门火衰而致的阳痿、早泄或疮疡久溃不敛等。

B.5　隔椒饼灸

用白胡椒末加面粉和水，制成直径2~3cm、厚0.5~0.8cm的薄饼。饼的中心放置药末（丁香、肉桂、人工麝香等）少许，然后置于应灸腧穴部位或患处，再将艾炷放在椒饼上点燃施灸。当艾炷燃尽，易炷再灸，直至灸完应灸的壮数。此法多用于治疗风湿痹痛及局部麻木不仁。

B.6　隔豉饼灸

用黄酒将淡豆豉末调和，制成直径2~3cm、厚0.5~0.8cm的薄饼，中间以针刺数孔，然后置于应灸腧穴部位或患处，再将艾炷放在豉饼上点燃施灸。当艾炷燃尽，易炷再灸，直至灸完应灸的壮数。此法多用于治疗痈疽发背初起，或溃后久不收口。

附　录　C

（资料性附录）

常用温灸器

C.1　灸架

　　灸架是一种特制的圆桶形或梯形塑料或木制灸具，四面镂空，顶部中间有一放置和固定艾条的圆孔，灸架内中下部距底边 3 ~ 4cm 安装铁窗纱一块，灸架两边有一底衽，另配有一根橡皮带和一灭火管。施灸时，将艾条点燃后插入孔中，以可上下自由移动为度，再将灸架固定在某一穴位上，用橡皮带套在灸架两边的底衽上，即可固定而不脱落；升降艾条调节距离，以微烫而不疼痛为适中。灸治完毕，将剩余艾条插入灭火管中（图 C1 ~ C3）。

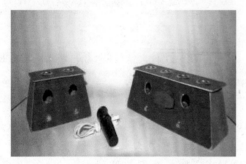

图 C1　梯形灸架

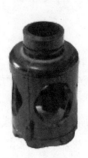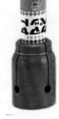

图 C2　桶形灸架

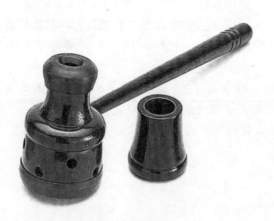

图 C3　带手柄灸架

C.2　灸筒

　　灸筒由内筒和外筒两部分相套而成，均用 2 ~ 5cm 厚的铁片或铜片制成。内筒和外筒的底、壁均有孔，外筒上用一活动顶盖扣住，内筒安置一定的架位，使内筒与外筒的间距固定。外筒上安置有一手柄便于把持。点燃放入内筒的艾绒,将内筒放回外筒,盖上顶盖,即可使用(图C4)。

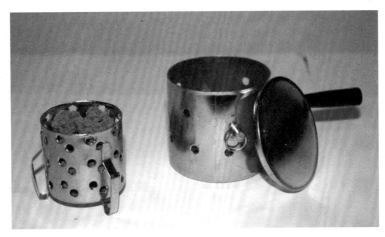

图 C4　灸筒

C.3　灸盒

灸盒是一种特制的木制长方形的盒形灸具。灸盒下面无底,上面有一可随时取下的与灸盒外径大小相同的盒盖,灸盒内中下部距底边 4～6cm 安装铁窗纱一块。施灸时把灸盒安放丁施灸部位,将点燃的艾绒或艾条置于铁纱上,盖上盒盖即可(图C5)。

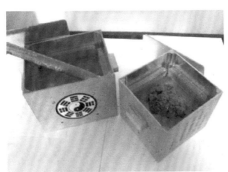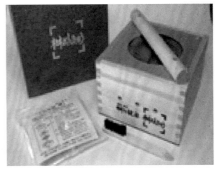

图 C5　灸盒

C.4　艾炷熏灸器

艾炷熏灸器是一种特制的金属圆形灸具,中空,下面无底,灸盒直径约 6cm,高约 2cm,顶部金属面上有若干置放和固定艾炷的小圆孔。施灸时,将若干艾炷插入孔中后点燃,手持艾盒或把艾盒安放于施灸部位(图C6)。

C.5　纸板灸

用宽 4～10mm、长 7～12mm 的纸将艾绒卷起,制作成直径 15～35mm、厚 2～5mm、正中心有小通风孔的硬纸板。将艾灸卷垂直固定在纸板中心。在进行治疗时,用黏附剂将纸板底部与皮肤相黏。胶水同样会阻止灰烬掉落,进而灼伤皮肤。纸板中心的通风孔会将热量传递。热量强度可以通过调节纸板厚度或艾灸卷的直径及等级来控

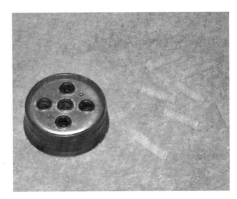

图 C6　艾炷熏灸器

制（图 C7 ~ C8）。

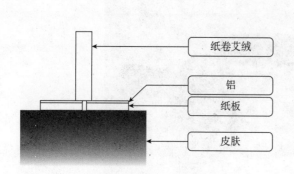

图 C7　纸板灸示意图

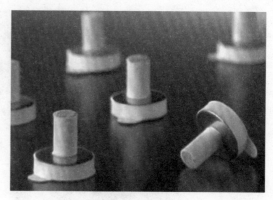

图 C8　纸板灸

C.6　艾管灸

将 0.1g 艾绒置于直径 7 ~ 10mm、高 10 ~ 15mm 纸管的顶部。用黏附剂将纸管底部与皮肤相黏。胶水同样会阻止灰烬掉落，进而灼伤皮肤。在艾绒点燃之后，热量将会通过管道传递到皮肤。艾绒产生的热量可以通过纸管的直径和合适等级的艾绒进行控制（图 C9 ~ C10）。

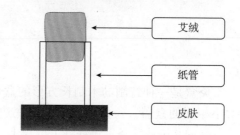

图 C9　艾管灸示意图

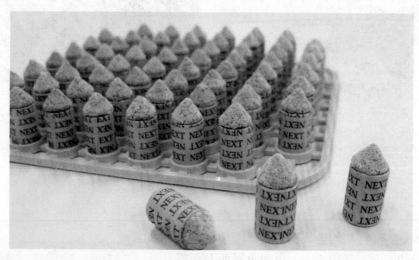

图 C10　艾管灸

C.7　灸碗或灸盘

灸碗或灸盘是指陶瓷圆形碗或盘，当点燃艾绒时会被加热。灸碗有一个盖子，盖上有小孔。灸盘没有盖子。热量强度根据陶瓷的厚度而有所不同，并且可以由铺垫在灸碗或灸盘与皮肤之间的棉布或纱布的层数而上升或下降（图 C11）。

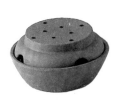
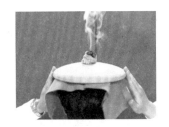

图 C11　灸碗和灸盘

C.8　灸缸

灸缸是指木柄、金属尖端的轻便型艾灸器材，小巧轻便。将燃烧的香艾条或清艾条从木柄处放入灸缸中，将其固定于某一特定点，使其不会到达金属尖端的底部。将灸缸放置在皮肤上，若有需要，可在两者之间加放数层纱布或棉布，以调节热度。结束治疗后，将灸缸倒置，取出艾条，灭火。某些灸缸可由陶器或其他金属制成（图 C12）。

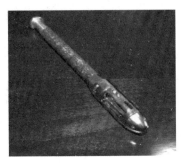
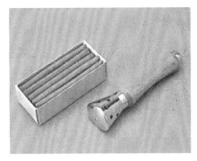

图 C12　灸缸和香艾条

附录 D

（规范性附录）

艾灸量、治疗时间及疗程

D.1 艾灸量

艾灸量是指艾灸治疗时所用的艾量，以及局部达到的温热程度。不同的灸量产生不同的治疗效果。艾炷灸的灸量是以艾炷的大小和壮数的多少计算，炷小、壮数少则量小，炷大、壮数多则量大；艾条温和灸、温灸器灸则以施灸的时间计算，时间越长，灸量越大；艾条实按灸是以点按皮肤的次数计算，点按次数越多，灸量越大。

D.2 艾炷的常见规格

根据艾炷的大小不同，温度也有所不同。一般而言，一个极小的艾炷和线一样细；小型艾炷直径 2 ~ 5mm，高 4 ~ 8mm；中型艾炷直径 6 ~ 10mm，高 9 ~ 13mm；大型艾炷直径 11 ~ 15mm，高 14 ~ 25mm（图 D1）。

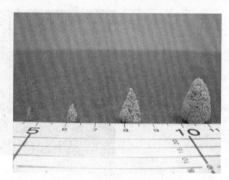

图 D1　艾炷的常见规格

D.3 针对不同部位、疾病及患者自身情况的艾灸量

一般而言，艾灸量由艾灸的不同部位、疾病、患者自身情况而决定。

在头面胸部、四肢末端皮薄而多筋骨处施灸，灸量宜小；在腰腹部、肩及两股等皮厚而肌肉丰满处施灸，灸量可大。

病情如属沉寒痼冷、阳气欲脱者，灸量宜大；若属外感、痈疽、痹痛，则应适度，以灸量小为宜。

凡体质强壮者，灸量可大；久病、体质虚弱、老年和小儿患者，灸量宜小。

D.4 艾灸治疗时间及疗程

每次施灸时间为 10 ~ 40 分钟，依疾病辨证确定。艾灸 5 ~ 15 次可为一个疗程。根据疾病类型和患者情况，两次瘢痕灸之间要间隔 1 ~ 10 天。

附　录　E

（规范性附录）

晕灸的处理办法

发生晕灸后，应立即停止艾灸，使患者头低位平卧，注意保暖，轻者一般休息片刻，或饮温开水后即可恢复；重者掐按水沟、内关、足三里穴即可恢复；严重时按晕厥处理。如果症状没有缓解，有必要寻求专业医生的帮助。艾灸师在进行上述操作时必须遵循自己所在国家的相关规定。

———————————